The Ultimate Cures And Remedies For Asthma

The Most Effective, Permanent Solution To Finally Cure Asthma

John K.

Table of Contents

Introduction

I want to thank you and congratulate you for purchasing the book, *"The Ultimate Cures and Remedies for Asthma"*.

This book contains proven steps and strategies on how to keep asthma under control.

While the respiratory condition isn't among the top causes of death or even prolonged hospitalization, it isn't a problem that you should overlook. If left unchecked, asthma could prove to be fatal, especially when coupled with respiratory infections. In other words, if you fail to keep asthma under control, a mere case of flu or cold could put you in a lethal situation. Well, there's no need to worry since you've got your hands on this book. Once you're done reading this, you'll know how to put an end to your respiratory concern. You'll know that taking medications and making lifestyle changes, among other things, could solve your problems.

Thanks again for purchasing this book, I hope you enjoy it!

Chapter 1: What is Asthma?

Asthma is a condition wherein the airways begin to narrow, swell, and then produce extra mucus. This condition can make breathing quite difficult; it can even trigger coughing, shortness of breath, and wheezing.

There are some people who consider asthma as minor nuisance but for others, asthma can be a huge problem that interferes with the activities they do every single day. Some even face life-threatening asthma attacks.

Asthma is one condition that cannot be cured, but its symptoms can be controlled. It is of utmost importance that you work well with your doctor to monitor your signs and your symptoms since asthma often changes through time and that translates to changes in your treatment as well.

The symptoms of asthma can range from minor to severe. Symptoms also differ from one person to the other. A person can have infrequent attacks or a person can develop those symptoms only during certain situations, or a person can have the symptoms of asthma all the time.

The commons signs and symptoms of asthma include any or all of the following:

> ➢ When you experience shortness of breath

> ➢ When you experience pain or tightness in your chest

> ➢ When you are having trouble sleeping because of your shortness of breath, coughing, wheezing, or a combination of the three

> ➢ When you can hear a whistling or wheezing sound every single time you exhale

> ➢ When your coughing or your wheezing is easily worsened by a respiratory illness like having a cold or having the flu

There are also severe signs of asthma which include any or all of the following:

> The asthma symptoms you experience occur more frequently and become more bothersome

> You are experiencing an increasing difficulty in breathing

> You need to use an inhaler more often

There are people whose asthma can be triggered by certain events like:

> Exercise: The asthma attack these people experience tend to worsen when the air is cold and dry

> Occupation: These people experience an attack when they are exposed to certain chemical fumes, gases in their surroundings, or even dust particles

> Allergy: The asthma attack of these people are triggered by certain allergens, like pet dander

It is very much advisable for you to seek the help of your doctor:

> …if you think you have developed asthma or you think that you have it, and if you have noticed that during the last few days or more you have been frequently coughing and wheezing. It is best to treat asthma in its early stages since that would prevent you from having long-term lung damage and early treatment would also prevent your asthma from becoming worse over time.

> …to help you monitor your asthma after you have been properly diagnosed with it. The best pal to be on your side when it comes to controlling the symptoms of your asthma would be your doctor. Great long-term care can help you feel better every single day and can prevent you from having a life-threatening asthma attack.

> …if you notice that your asthma is becoming worse. You must call your doctor right away if you notice that your current medications or

treatments do not ease your symptoms anymore, or if you have noticed that you are using your inhaler more frequently. You should never ever think about self-medicating. It would be wise for you to remember that when you overuse your asthma medication, you can from suffer serious side effects and that can make your asthma worse than it already is.

> To check on your treatment. Asthma is a condition that often changes as time passes by and meeting with your doctor on a regular basis is best since you can talk about your current symptoms and if there need to be certain adjustments when it comes to your medication.

When a person is having an asthma attack, the walls of that person's airways become inflamed and then the lining of the airways begin to secrete excessive amounts of mucus. Thus, when all this is happening, that person experiences difficulty breathing. As a result, that person may end up coughing a lot and wheezing a lot too.

Asthma attacks in people are triggered by different kinds of things like:

- ➢ Pollen

- ➢ Pets

- ➢ Molds

- ➢ Dust Mites

- ➢ Gastro esophageal reflux disease (GERD)

- ➢ Breathing in cold or dry air

- ➢ Exercise

- ➢ Smoke from tobacco

The symptoms of asthma tend to get much worse when the person also has a cold, the flu, or any other respiratory infection. There are also people who get attacks when they inhale certain chemicals, but sometimes people who have asthma experience an attack for no apparent reason at all.

Any person who has asthma faces the risk of having an attack, but that risk may be increased by certain things like: previous severe asthma attacks, being rushed to the hospital because of an attack, using up more than two inhalers in a month, attacks which tend to be sudden and unpredictable, and other health conditions like having sinusitis or having a nasal polyp.

Asthma should not be taken for granted since it can become quite serious, especially when attacks tend to interrupt your daily activities, like your sleeping habits, your school or work, and your exercise routine. It has the capacity to have quite a significant impact on your life and it often tends to be disruptive. You can even experience being brought to the emergency room just so you can be given aid in your breathing. Asthma in severe cases can lead to respiratory arrest and even death. You should not brush your asthma aside. If you think you have it go to your doctor now.

Chapter 2: What to Expect from Your Doctor

Before going to your doctor, it would be best if you are well-prepared so that you would be able to get most out of the time you have in your appointment. It is best if you try to do the following things:

> ➢ You must take your very own asthma action plan with you. If you do not have one yet, it would be best if you make one now. An asthma action plan is something that discusses how your asthma attacks are being treated.

> ➢ The results of your peak flow meter must be written down so that you can show it to your doctor as well.

> ➢ It would be very much helpful if you would list down all your medications so that your doctor can see all the medications you are taking.

> You must also be prepared to disclose with your doctor the symptoms you have been experiencing and how much your asthma attacks have been bothering you. These pieces of information and dates are very important since asthma is a condition which changes through time and that would most probably need a treatment that changes periodically.

> You must also be prepared to show your doctor how you are using your metered-dose inhaler since improperly using your inhaler can reduce its effectiveness and you would be using more of it.

Now that you are well-equipped with the information necessary for your appointment with your doctor, you must prepare the things you would like to ask your doctor. Here are a few questions which would be helpful to ask during your appointment so that no time would be wasted:

> Asking if you're current medications or your current treatment plan needs to be altered.

➢ You can also ask what signs you are going to experience if you are about to have an asthma attack.

➢ The measures you can do to avoid asthma attack, especially when your symptoms seem worse or when you are exposed to your asthma attack triggers.

➢ The medication you must take or the measures you must do in order for you to stop an asthma attack that is in progress.

➢ The instances when you should go to the emergency room.

➢ The measures you can do so that you can improve your immune system during cold or flu season.

You should not hesitate in asking other questions you might want answered by your doctor since these questions concern your health.

You now know what questions you are going to ask your doctor and you must be prepared for the questions your doctor might ask you, and here are some of those queries:

- ➤ If your asthma has worsened recently

- ➤ The medications you are taking

- ➤ The dosage of your medication

- ➤ The way you use your inhaler

- ➤ Problems you have encountered with your current medication

- ➤ Your asthma action plan

- ➤ Problems with your asthma action plan

- ➤ The things you cannot do because of your asthma

There are some tests that can be done on you, especially if you are an adult, so that the functionality of your lungs is determined. You asthma is not being properly controlled when you have poor lung function. These functions tests are most often utilized to check the severity of the asthma attack or to check how well the treatment administered is working for the patient.

These lung function tests can by any of the following:

➢ Peak flow

o During an asthma attack your doctor may take a peak flow reading on your scheduled appointment or when you seek for emergency medical care for your attack. This test determines how rapidly you can blow out. This test is very much helpful at home since you can monitor your own lung function and disclose any info you gather to your doctor during your appointments.

o This test is executed by allowing you to blow into a

mouthpiece as fast and as hard as you can, with one single breath. The result of this peak flow test is termed as your peak expiratory flow.

> Spirometry

o You are asked to take deep breaths and then to forcefully exhale through a hose which is connected to a spirometer. This test determines how much air you can breathe out in a single second. It can also measure the rate of your inhalations and exhalations, as well as how much air your lungs can hold. The result of this test is known as your forced expiratory volume.

> Nitric Oxide Measurement

o This is a new diagnostic test which aims to measure the amount of nitric oxide gas in your breath. When the nitric oxide in your breath is high, it means your bronchial tubes are quite inflamed.

- o This test requires you to slowly exhale into a mouthpiece which is attached to an electronic monitoring device. The device is connected to a computer which monitors your results.

- ➢ Pulse Oximetry

  - o This is a test done during severe asthma attacks since it measures the amount of oxygen in your blood. It is quite easy to do because a small device is clipped onto your finger and the results are shown through such device.

Chapter 3: Available Treatments and Drugs

A person having an asthma attack should follow the well-prepared asthma action plan he/she has worked out with his/her doctor. If that person's condition does not improve even if the necessary steps outlined in such action plan are taken, then that person should seek the help of a medical professional immediately.

Usually a person takes 2.5 to 5 milligrams of albuterol as part a home treatment plan. The albuterol is taken every twenty minutes for an hour. There are also people who take certain quick-acting medications. When it comes to treating children and adults with less severe symptoms of asthma, less medication is often given. A home treatment may also include certain oral corticosteroids, like prednisone.

An inhaler is best used when the result of your peak flow readings begin to deviate by 50 to 80 points from your usual results. It would be helpful it you are routinely checking you peak flow readings so that you can determine if a change has occurred in the results and thus, you can easily tell if your asthma is worsening or if an attack is about to happen.

Executing your asthma action plan is a basic thing to do for a person who is having an asthma attack. If the plan works then well and good, that person must continue following it. It gets quite tricky when the action plan does not give the desired results, such as relieving the symptoms of asthma experienced by the person. If that happens, the help of a doctor is required, making changes in the action plan so that it would work again. Once the doctor has determined the problem in your current action plan, your medication will probably be changed

or you'd be asked to avoid certain asthma triggers that you did not use to have. In those instances where your asthma attack has progressed so quickly that you can no longer wait to schedule an appointment with your doctor; you need to go to the emergency room so that you can be given immediate help.

In emergency cases, you can expect to be given the following medications:

> Short-acting beta agonists

o You are given this medication through a nebulizer which turns the medicine into a fine mist that you are to inhale so that your asthma symptoms are alleviated. The content of this medication is the same as that in your inhaler.

➤ Oral Corticosteroids

- o This medication is in pill form and this helps decrease the inflammation in your bronchial tubes, thus getting the symptoms of your asthma under control. For people with severe asthma this medication is given intravenously.

➤ Ipratropium

- o This medication is used to dilate the bronchial tubes of a person so that the symptoms of severe asthma can be treated. This medication is usually resorted to when the albuterol is not effective anymore.

➤ Intubation, mechanical ventilation, and oxygen

- o Once asthma attacks become life-threatening, a breathing tube is inserted into the patient's throat and a machine

is used to pump oxygen into
the lungs to help the patient
breathe. The tube stays in
while the medication for
asthma works its way into the
system of the patient. This is
the most extreme measure
that can be done.

Those are the things that may or may not
happen to you, once you enter the emergency
room. It all depends on how severe your attack
is. After the necessary medication is given to
you in the emergency room, the doctor will ask
you to stay there for a few hours to make sure
that you will not have another attack. Once the
doctor determines that you are no longer going
to have another attack soon, you will be asked
to go home and you are given the necessary
precautions and instructions.

If the doctor on the other hand determines that
your condition has not improved, you will be
asked to stay in the hospital for the next few
days so that your condition could be monitored
better and that you could be given the
necessary medications. If your symptoms are
quite severe, you can be asked to wear an
oxygen mask during the duration of your stay
in the hospital. For some people with severe
and persistent asthma, they are asked to stay in
the intensive care unit of the hospital since
their condition can be life-threatening.

There are numerous natural asthma remedies that can be utilized by anyone who has asthma. Here are some of these remedies:

- ➢ Herbs and dietary supplements

  - o There are a lot of herbs and supplements that can be used with asthma but these are not usually recommended since there has been no definite sign that they do help alleviate the condition.

- ➢ Yoga

  - o There are times when stress can trigger asthma and the breathing exercises in yoga are said to have helped people with asthma control their breathing and lessen their stress as well, which in turn weakens stress as a trigger for asthma attacks and symptoms.

- ➢ Asthma Diet

  - o If you have food allergies, you must avoid them so that your attacks would become less frequent as well.

➤ Acupuncture

- o There is not enough studies to prove that it reduces asthma attacks and that it improves breathing

➤ Biofeedback

- o If you can control your heart rate, that would be helpful in controlling and managing your asthma; however, not enough research has been done on this yet to conclusively state such.

There are natural remedies but their effectiveness and safety has not been fully tested and studied, so it would be wise to consult with your doctor first before taking anything or doing anything so that your health and safety can be ensured.

Chapter 4: Lifestyle Changes

Most of the time, avoiding an attack is all about managing your asthma with certain simple changes in your lifestyle.

- ➢ Exercise and Sports

    - o A person with asthma can exercise although that person has to ensure that his asthma is under control, otherwise his/her symptoms would just worsen when he engages in sports or exercises. It would be wise to talk to your doctor about this so that the both of you can make an asthma action plan that would be fit for you even if you exercise or engage in sports. You will know if the action plan is working if your asthma is still under control even if you're engaging in sports or exercising.

    - o If your asthma is well under control but you experience asthma symptoms five or ten minutes after you exercise, then you have exercise-induced asthma. This type of asthma happens when the airways of a person are very much sensitive to the temperature and the humidity changes around him/her. Whenever that persons breaths in cold and dry air through the mouth, asthma is triggered. The factors that affect exercise-induced asthma are:

- The duration of your exercise

- The weather outside

- The humidity of your surroundings

- The allergens in the air like

  - Pollution

  - Pollen

- Dust particles

o If you are not sure whether your symptoms are caused by the exercise or if your asthma is simply not under control, then you must talk to your doctor. After you and your doctor have already established an exercise regimen for you, it would be best that you remember these things:

  - You should take your medication before exercising if that is what your doctor told you.

  - Start slowly. You must take your time before you attempt to do more demanding exercise programs.

  - You must always warm up and cool down when you exercise.

- If you develop symptoms while you are exercising you must stop, take a break, and take your reliever medication.

- If you are used to exercising outside and it is cold out, exercise inside instead.

- If you are used to exercising outside and you have noticed that the pollen count is quite high or the pollution has worsened, you must exercise indoors instead.

- Keep in mind that the benefits of exercise far outweigh the risks that go with it since…

  - It can boost the efficiency of your heart and your lungs

- It can increase the strength of your muscles and your endurance

- It can improve your flexibility and your posture

- It can boost your ability to relax

➢ Pets and other animals

  o If a person is allergic to pets then that can definitely make their asthma worse.

  o There are certain animals that can trigger asthma like:

    - Cats

    - Gerbils and Hamsters

    - Dogs

- Mice, guinea pigs, and rats

- Rabbits

- Horses

- Birds

- The particles of the skin or dander, the oil secretions, the saliva, the feces and the urine of these animals are what you are sensitive to.

- If you're not willing to give away your beloved pet, it would be best to minimize your exposure to the allergens that it releases by:

  - Bathing it at least twice a week

  - Removing the carpeting in your home, especially in the bedrooms

- Cleaning the house with a vacuum equipped with a high-efficiency air filter or by using a central vacuum system with an outdoor exhaust

- Use special allergen-proof covers for your pillows and your mattresses

- Not allowing your pet to enter your bedroom

- Smoking

  - The smoke from tobacco triggers your asthma symptoms. It may be secondhand smoke or even firsthand smoke, but all the same it should be avoided since it is dangerous, especially for people with asthma.

- Pollution and other outdoor triggers

    - Every time you are outdoors you cannot control your surroundings and thus, you can have no control over your asthma triggers; but that does not mean that you cannot eliminate or reduce your exposure to these triggers. You can make a few adjustments and you can breathe better whenever you are outside.

    - Moulds

        - For many people, moulds are an asthma trigger. It is a fungus which has spores that float in the air and then inhaled by people which can cause the person to cough, to wheeze and even to experience tightness in the chest.

        - There are moulds in places which are damp like places with vegetation, places with garbage containers and

places with stagnant
water.

- If you are a person who
  is quite sensitive to the
  spores of moulds then
  you should try doing
  these things:

  - Remove the
    piles of grass on
    your lawn
    immediately
    after the grass is
    cut

  - Remove the
    leaves in your
    lawn

  - Make sure that
    the garbage cans
    in your house is
    clean

  - Remove the
    outdoor
    containers
    which hold
    water

- You must make sure that the eaves troughs on your house is facing away from your house

- o Pollen

  - This is quite a common trigger for asthma attacks and symptoms. It is airborne which means it can be easily inhaled by any person, especially during the months with warm weather. It is released by trees, grass, and even weeds.

  - If you are a person who is allergic to pollen, you must:

    - Utilize a HEPA-filtered air cleaner

    - Only plant low-allergen plants in your garden

- Use the air conditioner in your home and in your car; close your windows as much as possible during those months when the pollen count is quite high.

- Do not go out of the house between 5 to 10 in the morning during hot and windy days

- Try exercising inside when the pollen count outside is through the roof

- If you have been outside, change your clothes the moment you get in; and it would be best if you showered as well

- Remove plants in your yard which have high pollen content

- Use the dryer instead of hanging your clothes outside during those months when the pollen levels is quite high

- Cold Air

  o Any abrupt change in the weather can trigger your asthma symptoms.

  o If you are a person affected by cold weather, it would be best if you:

    - Breathe through your nose so that the air warms up before it reaches your lungs

    - Wear a mask or a scarf to help humidify the air

> you breathe through your mouth

- Exercise inside your home

➢ Air Pollutants

- These can worsen your symptoms, so it would be best if you:

  - Lessen your time in very polluted places

  - Exercise inside your house instead

  - Use the air conditioner in your home and in your car; close the windows

➢ Indoor triggers

- Dust Mites

  - Being allergic to dust mites is a problem for people with asthma since the excretions and the body parts of these creatures can be quite a strong trigger for asthma symptoms.

- For you to be able to minimize dust mites, you must:

    - Use a dehumidifier in damp areas

    - Remove carpets

    - Launder your bed linens in hot water

    - Use mite-allergen casings for your pillows and mattresses

- Cockroaches

    - The feces of these insects can trigger asthma attacks and symptoms.

o You must make sure that food and water are not in places where these creatures can reach them.

➢ Indoor Molds

o The best way to avoid these molds would be to keep your home dry and clean by:

- Monitoring humidity levels and using a dehumidifier

- Making sure that your home is well-ventilated

- Removing the carpets

- Cleaning moldy areas

- Ensuring that your house has a proper drainage

- Use fans in the kitchen and in the bathroom

- Decrease the number of plants in your home

➢ Chemical Fumes

o You must control exposure to these chemicals which can come in the form of paint or any other volatile products in your home.

Every asthma attack requires the use of a quick-acting inhaler, such as albuterol, but one of the key steps in avoiding an asthma attack would be to avoid its triggers. You can minimize your exposure to your asthma triggers by conducting an allergy test or by simply observing what seems to be triggering your asthma attacks at home, at school, or at work. It would also be very helpful for you to frequently wash your hands to avoid catching a cold or the flu, so that you would not suffer from both an attack and a respiratory infection. If your asthma seems to be triggered by cold air and you wish to exercise, it would be best to wear a mask or cover your face with a scarf until you are all warmed up.

Chapter 5: Prevention is the Best Cure

The best possible way for you to prevent a life-threatening asthma attack would be to make sure that your asthma is under control, meaning you need to have an action plan. You may not completely eliminate your risk of having an asthma attack but you are less likely to have one if your current treatment is keeping your respiratory system in the best shape possible. You must make sure that you are taking your medications as prescribed by your doctor, or as indicated in your asthma action plan.

The medication you are required to take on a daily basis treats the chronic inflammation in your airways which causes your asthma attacks. You must make sure that you take them every single day so that you can eliminate your asthma flare-ups and at the same time, decrease your need to use an inhaler.

If you are following your action plan but you have noticed that you are still being bothered by your symptoms and no relief is given to you by your medication, then it is time for you to give your doctor a call since this is a sign that your asthma is no longer under control. Simply put, you need to see your doctor so that a change in your action plan can be made, together with a change in your current treatment.

When you have a cold or the flu, keep track of how you're feeling. Don't forget to take your asthma medications as well as your vitamins. If you fail to do that, you might suddenly find it harder to breathe. Also, be sure to steer clear of allergens. As pointed out in the previous chapter, allergens do nothing but aggravate your symptoms and worsen your condition. During cold season it would be wise to have a mask handy so that the air would not bother you whenever you go out.

Basically, all you've learned from this book up to this point should be used in a preventive sense. Know the things that could be detrimental to your respiratory health and be sure to stay away from them.

Chapter 6: Asthma Action Plan

As emphasized a number of times in the previous chapters, one of the best ways for you to avoid attacks and to avoid developing symptoms would be to follow an effective action plan.

An asthma action plan is a program made specifically for you. It exists to help you manage your asthma. It is something you must create together with your doctor. It is a strategy that you can utilize to manage your asthma whenever it gets out of control. As with any important plan, it's most effective when written down. Despite being personalized, all action plans make use of zones.

You are in the green zone if your asthma is well under control. You are in the yellow zone if your asthma is not totally controlled and this means that you are in need of an adjustment when it comes to your medication. You are in the red zone whenever you are experiencing severe symptoms of asthma, meaning that your asthma is completely out of control – you need immediate medical attention.

Your action plan tells you when you are in
these zones, and makes it clear what you must
do whenever you reach either of the two danger
zones.

Conclusion

Thank you again for purchasing this book!

I hope this book was able to help you learn more about asthma, particularly when it comes to matters regarding causes and treatments.

The next step is to apply what you've learned firsthand, or share the info that you've gained with those who need it the most.

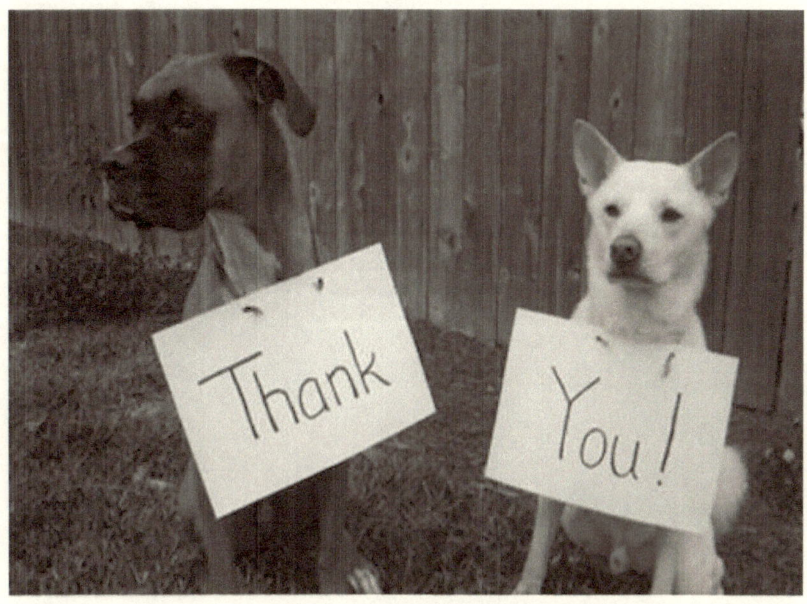

Finally, if you enjoyed this book, then I'd like to ask you for a favor, would you be kind enough

to leave a review for this book on Amazon? It'd
be greatly appreciated!

Thank you and good luck!

Check Out My Other Books

Below you'll find some of my other popular books that are popular on Amazon and Kindle as well. Simply click on the links below to check them out. Alternatively, you can visit my author page on Amazon to see other work done by me. If the links do not work, for whatever reason, you can simply search for these titles on the Amazon website to find them.

1) The Ultimate Guide To Overcome Anger - How To Manage Your Anger Before It Controls You

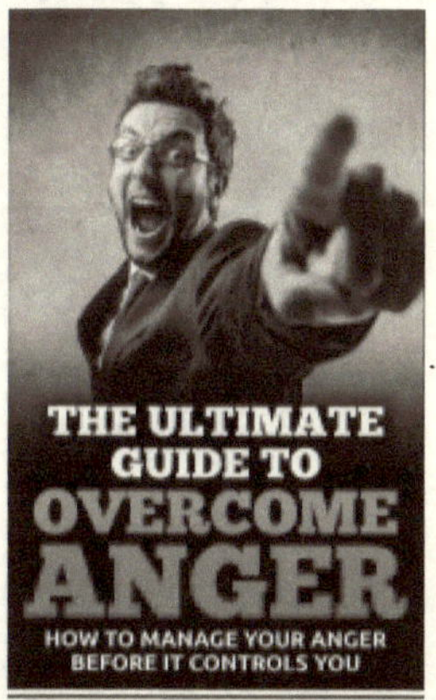

go to: http://amzn.to/1Pzm3Yy

2) The Ultimate Guide To Become An Alpha Male - How To Attract Women, Win In Life And Be Confident

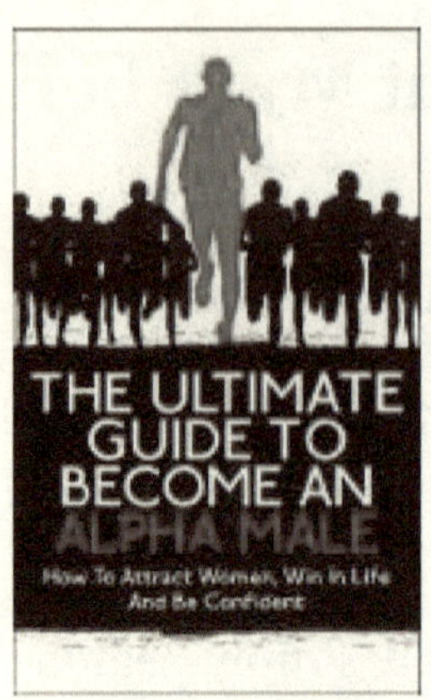

go to: http://amzn.to/20G8bBo

3) The Ultimate Guide To Overcome Porn Addiction For Life - The Most Effective, Permanent Solution To Finally Stop Porn Addiction

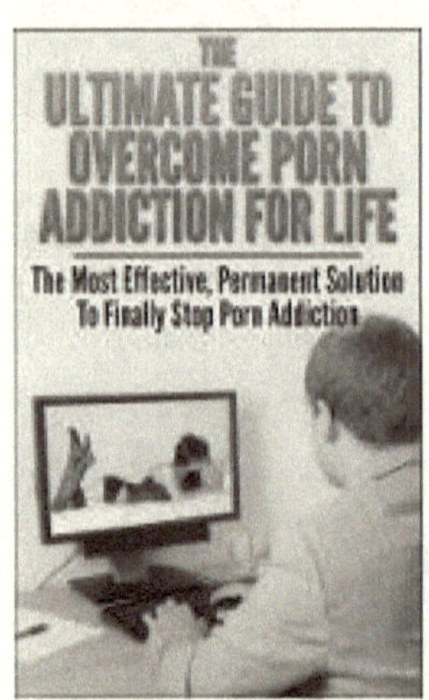

go to: http://amzn.to/1NZ2tmN

4) The Drug Addiction Cure - The Most Effective, Permanent Solution to Finally Overcome Drug Addiction for Life

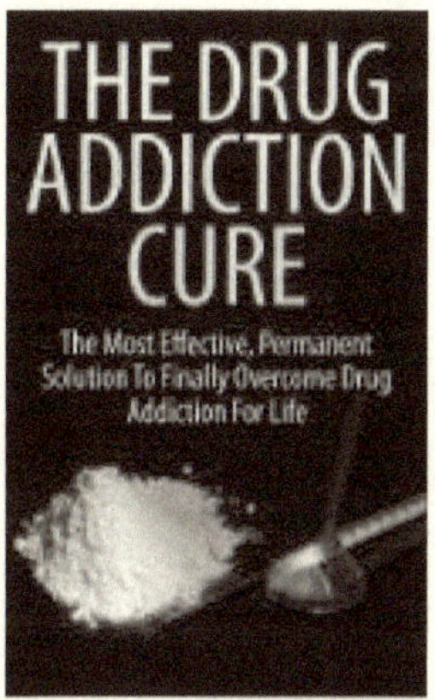

go to: http://amzn.to/1kkb9uc

5) How to Stop Snoring for Life - The Most Effective Cures and Remedies for Snoring

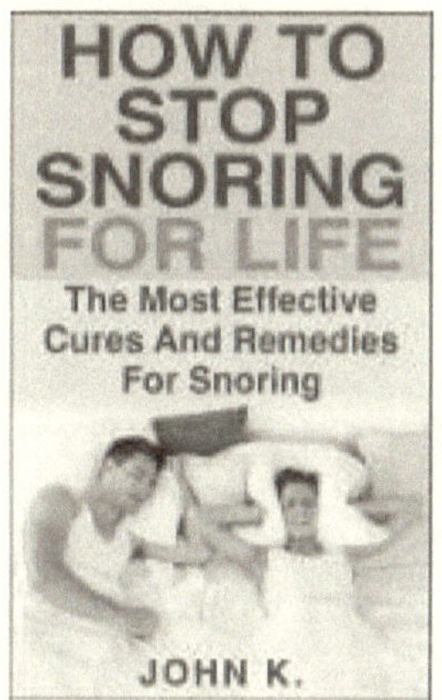

go to: http://amzn.to/1NE9uLn

www.ingramcontent.com/pod-product-compliance
Lightning Source LLC
Chambersburg PA
CBHW051126250726
48655CB00007B/2909